The Powerful Step-By-Step Guide To Reversing Diabetes

Table of contents

Introduction

Diabetes! I wouldn't be surprised if paranoia starts setting in upon hearing this term. All of us have a lot of questions every time we hear about a health disorder. I know, by now, your mind would have already started asking questions about diabetes. What is diabetes? What causes diabetes? How will I know if I am at a risk of developing diabetes? Is diabetes curable? Do I have to take medicines forever if I get diagnosed with diabetes? Can I reduce my risk factors with the help of a healthy diet?

Well, all your questions are definitely answered in this book. The aforesaid paranoia sets in because of our lack of knowledge about a particular thing. Being paranoid will definitely not help you if you get diagnosed with diabetes. Hence, it is important that you understand how diabetes works, considering how most of us are at the risk of developing diabetes.

You have done a great job by buying this book, as it is designed in such a manner that it equips you with all the basic information that you are required to know about diabetes. The first chapter is loaded with the answers to most of your questions regarding diabetes. The second chapter deals with tips to reverse/manage diabetes with the help of diet. The final chapter again contains some additional tips to effectively change your lifestyle to manage diabetes.

I am fairly positive that your knowledge on this disorder will improve by the end of this book. This knowledge will prepare you to deal with your risks better and manage diabetes, should you ever develop it. I hope you will find this book useful. Thank you for buying this book.

Chapter 1: Understanding Diabetes

When it comes to tackling any health issue, it is important that you have a thorough understanding about it. This knowledge will help you understand how your body functions, where you stand in terms of tackling the disorder/disease and effectively manage it. This is precisely why this chapter is designed to give you an overview about what diabetes is all about. I am sure you are not foreign to the term "diabetes". It has in fact become an overtly used word in the health sector because of the increasing risk that today's generation faces of suffering from it. This chapter will truly enhance your knowledge on the subject and help you gauge where you stand.

What is diabetes?

Diabetes is nothing but a disorder of our endocrine system by virtue of which, the blood sugar levels are higher than the normal range. Diabetes can be caused due to a variety of reasons and all these reasons are in a way related to the amount of insulin produced by our body and the way our body reacts to insulin.

Insulin is a hormone, which is produced by our pancreas. This helps our body in storing the fat and the sugar content present in the food that we consume every day. Typically, diabetes occurs when any of the following happens:

- ➢ When the pancreas stops producing any insulin.
- ➢ When the pancreas produces insulin, but in very minimal quantities.
- ➢ When the cells in our body stop responding to insulin in an appropriate fashion. This is also known as insulin resistance, which will be dealt a little later in this book.

Role of insulin in Diabetes

Preliminary understanding of how insulin works would help you in understanding its role in diabetes. Our body consists of millions and millions of cells. These cells require energy to function, for which they require food that is broken down into a very simple form. Whenever we consume something, the body breaks the food into a compound called "glucose", which in turn provides energy for the cells in our body. Insulin plays an important role in regulating the amount of glucose present in your blood. The pancreas always releases the hormone in small amounts. Whenever it senses that the glucose levels in your blood are increasing, it secretes more insulin to push the glucose into our cells. This will eventually bring down the glucose content in your bloodstream. Now, the converse also happens. Whenever the body feels that the glucose levels in your blood are low, it immediately signals you to eat and also releases glucose stored in your liver into the bloodstream.

As we saw earlier, people suffering from diabetes have issues with either the secretion of insulin or their body is resistant to insulin. Hence, these result in the glucose levels in the bloodstream go unmonitored and stay high.

Types of Diabetes

Yes, it is important that you are aware about the different types of diabetes as well, to understand the risks associated with each type.

Type I diabetes

As I mentioned before, insulin is produced by the pancreas. To be more precise, it is the beta cells present in the pancreas, which produce insulin. Type I diabetes is a phenomenon whereby these beta cells are destroyed by our immune system. Hence, people suffering from this type of diabetes produce no insulin. Their source of insulin is reduced to insulin injections, which will have to be administered regularly to monitor the blood sugar levels. This is most common in people, who are younger than 20 years old, but then people of all age groups stand the risk of getting this type of diabetes.

Type II diabetes

In this case, the body continues to produce insulin. However, the problem lies in the fact that the insulin produced is either not enough or the body has become resistant towards the effects of the insulin. When this happens, the glucose present in the blood does not find its way into the various cells. This is the most common type of diabetes.

While this type of diabetes can be prevented through diet, if left unchecked, this type of diabetes can lead to other types of health complications such as amputations, blindness, chronic kidney failure etc. This type of diabetes usually occurs in people who are generally over the age of 40. Being overweight also increases the risk of this type. However, in today's scenario, even children are at the risk of suffering from this type of diabetes because of the rise in obesity among children.

This type of diabetes can be easily prevented with the help of a proper diet and regular exercising.

Gestational diabetes

This type of diabetes is caused because of pregnancy. As you may know, there are hormonal changes that happen during pregnancy, which in turn may affect the functioning of insulin. Pregnant women who are above normal weight before pregnancy and over the age of 25 stand the risk of suffering from gestational diabetes.

Screening for this type of diabetes is usually done at the time of pregnancy itself. If left untreated, this diabetes can increase the risk of complications not just for the mother but also for the unborn child. In fact, the baby is at a greater risk than the mother in this case. Some of the risks faced by the baby includes but not limited to breathing problems at the time of birth, abnormal weight gain before the baby is born, obesity after birth and the risk of diabetes at a later point in time.

These are the different types of diabetes.

What are my risk factors?

The problem with diabetes is that it often goes undetected. This is precisely why you should look at the below risk factors to understand where you stand.

I. Type I Diabetes

Below are the risks associated with Type I diabetes:

- ➤ Diseases of the pancreas: this can affect the ability of the beta cells to produce insulin.
- ➤ Family history: If this type of diabetes runs in the family, it is better to be safe than sorry. Go for a blood test to check if you have got it as well.
- ➤ Illness or infection: There are a handful of diseases/infections that are capable of affecting the functioning of your pancreas.

II. Type II Diabetes:

Here are some of the risk factors associated with this type of diabetes:

- ➤ Impaired glucose tolerance: This can be easily diagnosed with the help of a blood test. If you have impaired glucose tolerance, then you have the risk of getting type II diabetes.
- ➤ Obesity or overweight: This is one of the important reasons for type II diabetes. Hence, if you are obese or overweight, it is necessary that you are on the lookout for this diabetes.
- ➤ Ethnic background: Alaska natives, Hispanic/Latino Americans, Native Americans, African Americans, Asian Americans and Pacific Islanders stand a greater risk of getting type II diabetes.
- ➤ Cholesterol levels: If your body has low levels of good cholesterol and high levels of triglycerides, you are at risk.
- ➤ High blood pressure: If you have hypertension, you are again at risk.
- ➤ Insulin resistance: This happens when your body stops reacting to the effects of insulin. In other words, this means extra work for your pancreas.
- ➤ Family history: If your parent or sibling has this type of diabetes, you are at risk too.
- ➤ Sedentary lifestyle: If you have a sedentary lifestyle, not only will it lead to obesity but it also increases your risk of getting type II diabetes.

> Age: If you are over 40 and overweight, you stand a chance of getting diabetes.
> Polycystic ovary syndrome: This is a risk that only women face. Women, who suffer from polycystic ovary syndrome, are at a risk of easily getting type II diabetes.

III. *Gestational Diabetes*

Here is the list of risks associated with gestational diabetes:

> Obesity or overweight: If you are obese or overweight, it is necessary that you are on the lookout for this diabetes when you are pregnant.
> Family history: If your mother or sister had gestational diabetes when they were pregnant, there is all likelihood that you may also get it when you are pregnant. Hence, keep an eye on the family history.
> Glucose intolerance: If you have had glucose intolerance in the past, you stand a chance of getting gestational diabetes.
> Medical history: If you had gestational diabetes the last time you got pregnant, the chances of you getting it again is very high.
> Age: The age at which you get pregnant also matters. The older you are when you get pregnant, the higher are your risks of getting gestational diabetes.

I hope this chapter helped you understand all the basics of diabetes. This knowledge will definitely help you deal with it in an efficient manner. Further, this knowledge will also help you appreciate the usefulness of the tips mentioned in the upcoming chapters.

Chapter 2: Reversing diabetes with diet

Now that you have fair idea about diabetes, let us look at some tips to deal with it by tweaking your diet. Contrary to popular belief, it is absolutely possible to deal with diabetes by merely controlling your diet. I am sure that this chapter will help you change your perspective about dealing with diabetes.

Opt to consume dairy products daily

Research shows that people who consumed low fat dairy products had lower risks of suffering from type II diabetes as opposed to other people who didn't consume dairy products. Several studies show that insulin secretion in our body is stimulated by certain milk proteins. Further, dairy products are also packed with nutrients such as calcium, magnesium and vitamin D, which are also instrumental in lowering the risk of diabetes. Another added advantage of consuming dairy products is that you will have less room for other junk foods or foods rich in carbohydrates (which may end up increasing your risk of getting diabetes). If you are a dairy hater, take it slow. Start with your breakfast. Let go of your bagel or muffin for breakfast. Instead, choose a glass of skim milk and consume it along with fresh fruits. Grab a bite of low fat string cheese to satisfy your hunger pangs.

A colorful meal

Research shows that if your diet is made of fresh produce, your risk of getting diabetes is substantially reduced. A latest research shows that adults who consumed a lot of vegetables and fruits had a 21% lower risk of suffering from type II diabetes, when compared with adults of the same age group who did not consume vegetables or fruits in large quantities. The key is to not just eat vegetables and fruits but eat different kinds of produce. It is the variety that reduces your risk more than the quantity consumed. Ensure that you include a vegetable or fruit in every meal.

Now why including fiber rich foods like fruits and vegetables is important? Here is a list of reasons, which will help you realize that consumption of fruits and veggies will definitely reduce your risk of diabetes:

> ➤ Consumption of fiber in large quantities is capable of directly improving your insulin sensitivity.
> ➤ Fiber slows down the digestive process, which means that the body is going to take longer to break the food into glucose. In other words, the release of glucose into your bloodstream will be slower than before. Hence, you will not have a sudden increase in your glucose levels after a heavy meal, rich in fiber. Your glucose metabolism process is also streamlined as a result of this.

> Increased intake of fiber rich foods will also help in suppressing the glucose production by the liver.
> Another added advantage of consuming fiber is that you will feel full easily. Moreover, you will feel less hungry between meals. Hence, the urge to consume junk foods in between your meals is drastically reduced. As we already know, junk foods are rich in sugars and are capable of increasing your risk of developing diabetes.
> A diet rich in fiber is capable of altering the way the bacteria in your gut function. It results in the microbes consuming more calories from your food, thereby ensuring that only fewer calories are passed to your body.
> A fiber rich diet will definitely help you in maintaining your health and weight as well. As we already saw, being overweight or obese increases your risk of getting types II diabetes (and also gestational diabetes, if you are a woman). Hence, it is highly important that you are not just health conscious but also weight conscious.

These are some of the ways by which a fiber rich diet decreases your risk of getting diabetes. Hence, make sure that you consume a lot of fresh produce every day.

Say no to white rice

A study conducted recently shows that people who consume white rice in large quantities stand a higher risk of developing diabetes than others. White rice contains magnesium, vitamins and fiber in minimal quantities. Further, white rice is regarded as a high glycemic food. This means that it gets digested easily by the body, which in turn will result in sudden spikes in the blood sugar levels. If you are a rice lover, try choosing brown rice. If you do not like the taste of brown rice, mix it with little white rice to begin with, till you get used to its flavor.

Increase your intake of omega 3 fatty acids

Eight out of ten diabetic people also suffer from heart complications and associated disorders and end up losing their lives. A common reason for such sudden heart attacks is the off rhythm heartbeats. A research conducted in Netherlands shows that people who suffer from diabetes as well as heart complications have the opportunity to cut down their risk of getting a cardiac arrest by increasing their intake of omega 3 fatty acids. Say yes to all kinds of foods that are rich in omega 3 fatty acids. Go for sardines, salmon, trout and mackerel, as they are loaded with omega 3 fatty acids. Similarly, go for walnuts, flaxseed, canola oil, pumpkin seeds, spinach, kale and salad greens.

Increase your protein intake

It is natural for us to crave for something sugary when we feel that our energy levels are dipping down. But then again, it is bad news to yield to our temptations and go for sugary treats. They are packed with carbohydrates and are empty calories. Allow me to introduce you to a nutrient, which will help you deal with your dropping energy levels –

Proteins! Proteins are capable of stimulating the cells in your brain and make you feel energized. Hence, the next time you feel drained or sluggish, do not reach out for a carb. Go for an egg or chicken, which are rich in protein content. These protein rich foods are not only easily available but are also capable of improving your health.

Say no to grains

As you may already know, grains such as wheat are high on gluten content. Moreover, these grains are also high in terms of carbohydrates content. Upon consumption, they are broken down into sugar by our digestive system within few minutes. This naturally results in a sudden spike in the blood sugar levels. Added to this is the problem of the gluten content in the grains. Gluten is capable of causing inflammation in the intestines, which in turn affects the secretion and functioning of hormones such as leptin and cortisol. This again has an impact on the level of sugar present in your bloodstream.

Let go of refined sugar

Consumption of foods, which contain refined sugar, is capable of impacting the blood sugar levels in a drastic fashion. Consumption of beverages, soda and packaged fruit juice is capable of releasing sugar into your bloodstream in a rapid fashion. This rapid entry causes sharp elevations in the blood sugar levels. This is again not good news for your body! Your risk of getting type II diabetes is considerably increased. Hence, steer away from foods that are loaded with refined sugar. Go for a healthier sweetener such as stevia. Go for fresh fruit juices instead of beverages or soda drinks.

Count on the chromium

Chromium is capable of increasing our body's glucose tolerance. It is also capable of balancing out the sugar levels present in the bloodstream. Hence, consuming foods rich in chromium is a smart move to deal with diabetes as well as reduce your risk of developing diabetes. Some examples of foods that are rich in chromium are raw cheese, grass fed beef, broccoli and green beans. However, research shows that broccoli contains the maximum amount of chromium, in comparison with other foods.

Keep an eye on what you drink

If you are someone who loves alcohol, this tip is more relevant for you. If you are already suffering from diabetes, one or two drinks a day is sufficient to do enough damage. This also is capable of affecting your vision. Further, the consumption of alcohol is also capable of increasing your blood sugar levels. Alcohol consumption will also lead to liver toxicity. Sweet liquors and beer are loaded with carbohydrates. Hence, it is highly important that you stay away from these drinks.

Be careful with your caffeine intake

Caffeine is capable of reacting in strange ways. People, who are not diabetic, can reduce their risk of developing diabetes by consuming coffee. The caffeine content present in the coffee is capable of reducing your risk, according to research. However, studies also show that caffeine acts in an opposite manner when it comes to diabetic people. A study showed that consumption of coffee by a diabetic person increased the sugar levels in the bloodstream by around 21%. The study also showed that the consumption of caffeine also resulted in insulin resistance by the body. In other words, your body will have trouble in absorbing the sugar present in your bloodstream because of the influence of the caffeine. Hence, if you are a diabetic, stay away from drinks high on caffeine. Go for healthier drinks such as herbal tea, water or decaf.

Have more salads and citrus fruits

Salads and citrus fruits are loaded with magnesium, fiber and polyphenols. These nutrients help the cells in your body remain sensitive to insulin. Hence, you can reduce the risk of developing type II diabetes by increasing your consumption of these foods. When it comes to diabetic people, consumption of these kinds of foods will help them deal with diabetes without consuming too much of medicines. Studies show that citrus fruits such as grapefruit and tangerines are loaded with compounds such as nobiletin and narigenin. These compounds are capable of dealing with insulin resistance.

Choose your fats wisely

Though certain fats are considered unhealthy, there are fats that are actually beneficial. Hence, it is important that you exercise caution while choosing fatty foods. Below is a gist of the different kind of fats, which will help you choose your foods in an appropriate fashion:

- **Healthy fats:** The healthiest fats are the unsaturated fats. Foods such as nuts, olive oil, avocados and fish are rich in unsaturated fats. These fats are capable of moderating the sugar levels present in your bloodstream. Moreover, foods like salmon and tuna are also rich in omega 3 fatty acids. The benefits of consuming foods rich in omega 3 fatty acids have already been mentioned earlier in this chapter.
- **Unhealthy fats:** The most dangerous fats are synthetic trans fats. These are made by incorporating hydrogen with liquid vegetable oils. This is primarily done by the food manufacturers to increase the shelf life of these oils. These are extremely bad for you. You tend to put on weight easily if you consume these kinds of fats on a prolonged basis. We have already seen that being overweight/obese will definitely increase your risk of developing type II diabetes. Further, if you are diabetic, not keeping an eye on your weight will definitely increase your risk of developing heart related problems. Hence, staying fit will not only help you prevent diabetes but also deal with diabetes in an efficient fashion (if you are already a diabetic person). So, the key is to bid goodbye to these unhealthy fats.

- **Saturated fats:** There is a common misconception that reducing the consumption of saturated fats will help you lose weight. However, what happens when you reduce the consumption of fats altogether is that you are forced to consume more carbohydrates. We have already seen how the increased consumption of carbohydrates has an impact on your blood glucose levels. Hence, the key is to limit the intake of saturated fats.

Hence, make sure that you choose your fats in a wise fashion. Some tips to include healthy fats in your meal and reduce the consumption of unhealthy fats are as follows:

- ➢ As much as possible, avoid frying your food. Choose healthier methods of cooking such as baking, broiling or stir frying.
- ➢ Let go of chips and crackers. Instead, opt for nuts and seeds as they are healthier options for snacks.
- ➢ If you intend to opt for red meat, go for organic or grass fed versions of it.
- ➢ Do not go for commercial salad dressings. These are not only high in terms of calories but are also loaded with trans fat. Hence, make your own salad dressings with the help of flaxseed oil or extra virgin olive oil or sesame oil.
- ➢ When it comes to using oil for cooking, use coconut oil if you are cooking something on the stove. Go for cold pressed extra virgin olive oil for making salads, pasta dishes and for cooking vegetables.
- ➢ Make sure that you include avocado as much as possible in your meal, be it as part of your sandwich or as guacamole.
- ➢ Go for raw or organic milk, butter, yogurt and cheese as much as possible.

Include cinnamon
Cinnamon is capable of controlling the sugar levels in your bloodstream. Hence, include at least 2 teaspoons of cinnamon daily as part of your meal. You may choose to add it to your tea or smoothie or as a seasoning to your main course.

Avoid packaged foods
Packaged and processed foods not only add pounds to your weight but also affect the functioning of the kidneys and the liver. This will in turn increase your risk of developing diabetes. Hence, avoid foodstuffs such as soy, canola oil, soybean oil, cottonseed oil and vegetable oil from your diet.

Go for high fiber and slow release carbohydrates
We have already seen the effects of carbohydrates on our blood glucose levels. The problem with most carbohydrates is that they are easily broken down by our body and sugar is released into the bloodstream too soon. However, there are certain foods rich in carbohydrates, which are also known as slow release carbs. These are digested in a very

slow fashion by the body. This ensures that your body does not produce too much insulin. Here is a list of foods that consist of slow release carbohydrates:

- Sweet potatoes
- Yams
- Brown rice
- Cauliflower rice
- Whole wheat pasta
- Cauliflower mash
- Whole grain bread
- Spaghetti squash
- Whole wheat bread
- Rolled oats
- High fiber and low sugar cereal
- Peas
- Low sugar bran flakes
- Leafy greens

Choose foods with low glycemic index

Foods that have high glycemic index are capable of spiking your blood sugar levels in a sudden fashion. Foods that have low GI will help you regulate your blood sugar levels. Here is a list of foods that generally have low GI:

- Beans
- Eggs
- Cheese
- Milk
- Raw nuts
- Fish oils
- Olive oil
- Avocado
- Flaxseed
- Fresh fruits
- Fresh vegetables
- Legumes
- High fiber cereals
- Shellfish
- Fish
- Free range chicken
- Turkey
- Unsweetened yogurt

I am sure that your confidence in dealing with diabetes would have tremendously improved. I am sure you will completely agree with me when I say that it is completely possible to take care of diabetes with the help of diet.

Chapter 3: Other tips to manage diabetes

Now that we have seen how diabetes can be reversed as well as managed through foods, here are some additional tips to help you deal with diabetes. These tips will help you handle the sudden change in your lifestyle, which is required to deal with diabetes.

Stay away from plastics

The presence of chemicals such as phthalates in our blood levels increases our risk of developing type II diabetes. These chemicals are found in a variety of products around us. These can be found in clothing, building materials, cosmetics, toys, food packaging, perfumes, personal care products and vinyl products. Though the exposure to these chemicals does not directly cause diabetes, these have the tendency to affect the production of insulin.

Although it is not possible to completely to avoid things laced with these chemicals, you can always reduce your exposure to the extent possible. Try avoiding plastic containers, which have the recycling symbol 3 written on the bottom. Go for beauty products that are free from phthalates. Reading the labels of these products will help you choose those that are safe. For instance, if the label of your cosmetic product mentions that "fragrance" is an added ingredient, then steer away from the product as this is an indication that it contains phthalates. Similarly, ensure that your house is nicely ventilated.

Read labels and avoid processed foods

If you already don't have the habit of reading labels, now is a good time to start doing it. You will be able to eliminate pretty much all of the unhealthy foodstuffs by reading the labels. When you read the labels, you will be able to able identify those goods that are high in terms of sugar and trans fat content. This will help you steer away from these products easily.

Similarly, avoid buying processed foods such as canned foods, frozen meals or low fat meals. These often have added sugar or fat content. Packaged foods have hidden sugar content, which definitely is bad news! How do you spot the hidden sugar content? Pretty simple – read the labels! Look out for any of the following terms – cane crystals, agave nectar, crystalline fructose, evaporated cane juice, corn sweetener, dextrose, fructose, maltose, high fructose corn syrup, lactose, invert sugar, malt syrup etc. These terms are interchangeably used for sugar and this indicates that the food has added sugar in it. These are highly unhealthy, which is why you should avoid them. Go for fresh or frozen vegetables and healthier alternatives.

Take the help of your family and friends

I know that the thought of following a diet and exercise schedule alone can be a daunting task. Don't worry. Learn to form a support group for yourself. Team up with your family, friends and doctor. This will definitely help you stay motivated and on the track to recovery. Keeping your family and friends in the loop will also ensure that they don't tempt you with foodstuffs that will either increase your risk of developing diabetes or your blood sugar levels. You will hardly find the diet difficult to follow if you have the support of your loved ones. Similarly, it is important that you get your doctor on board before you change your diet.

Make time for exercise

It is important that you make some time in your daily routine for exercising. This is because your fitness has a direct impact on your risk of developing diabetes. When I say exercise, I am not just talking about cardio. It should be a combination of both strength workouts and cardio exercises. Research shows that diabetic people who did a combination of aerobic exercises as well as strengthening exercises were able to regulate their sugar levels better than other diabetic people who lead a sedentary lifestyle. If you are a busy professional and don't really have a flexible schedule, just try to squeeze in fifteen minutes of exercise every day. You can opt to do cardio exercises for around five minutes and strengthening exercises for another ten minutes.

Being physically fit will definitely have a positive impact on your diabetes. When you work out your muscles automatically contract. When this contraction happens, sugar molecules are pumped into the different cells in your body. Hence, these sugar molecules leave your bloodstream when you work out. And this benefit will continue to last even hours after you have finished exercising. Hence, there is better sugar control when you exercise regularly. You will seldom experience a sudden spike in your blood sugar levels, when you work out regularly. This also reduces the risk of developing other complications associated with diabetes such as vision loss, kidney problems and nerve damage.

Regular exercise will also reduce your body's resistance to insulin. Hence, your risk of developing type II diabetes is considerably reduced.

Get enough sleep

Research shows that lack of sleep or inadequate sleep is capable of increasing a diabetic person's morning blood sugar by at least 23%. The same research shows that insulin resistance is also increased by around 82%. Sleeping habits have a direct impact on your blood sugar levels. Hence, ensure that you get enough sleep every day. If you don't feel fresh enough, even after getting enough sleep, don't go for a cup of coffee immediately. We have already seen the adverse effects of caffeine, if you are a diabetic person.

Instead, try drinking other healthier beverages or begin your workout early in the day. If you have trouble sleeping for a prolonged duration, get it checked with your doctor.

Set goals

I know that your world turns upside down when you are diagnosed with diabetes. You are expected to change your routine and eating habits out of the blue to effectively manage your diabetes. As overwhelming as it may sound, it is definitely possible for you to tackle diabetes in a phased manner. Start setting goals. The key is to take it slow. It is not possible for you to change your habits overnight. Begin with goals for the day. Try tackling your goals, one day at a time. Once you feel that you are gaining control over these changes to your routine, devise weekly goals. Similarly, come up with goals for the entire month. As you have seen in the previous chapter, it is completely possible to manage diabetes purely through diet. Once you get the hang of the diet, you will definitely be encouraged to follow this new lifestyle with lot more enthusiasm.

Don't get bogged down by pain

Studies show that close to half the number of people who suffer from diabetes also suffer from arthritis. When you suffer from arthritis, exercising would definitely add a lot of strain to your already paining joints. Do not give up just because the pain sets in. Remember that staying fit is really important for you to manage your diabetes in an effective fashion. If the pain exists for a long period, consult your doctor for getting his suggestions to follow your exercise schedule in an effective fashion, despite your medical condition.

Take care of your emotional health

Your stress levels also have an impact on your diabetes. It is important that you take care of your emotional health as well. Focusing just on treating your diabetes, while ignoring your mental health, can be quite detrimental to your overall wellbeing. Research shows that you can treat your diabetes as well as issues related to your mental health (such as depression) at the same time. This research also shows that you will be able to recover sooner if you undergo the treatment for both the medical conditions at the same time. However, it is important that you get in touch with your doctor first and understand the consequences of the treatments available to you and take an informed decision.

Have a food diary

Maintain a food diary. This will help you track your eating habits in an effective fashion. Keeping a food diary also has the following benefits:

> ➢ It will help you identify the problematic areas in your current diet. For instance, a food diary will help you track the intake of unhealthy fats. This awareness will

help you consciously cut down your intake of these foodstuffs loaded with unhealthy fats.

- ➢ It will also help you identify patterns in your eating. For instance, some of us have cravings for sweets post lunch. This will induce you to indulge in sugary treats without giving much thought to what you eat. This awareness will again help you identify unhealthy eating patterns and get rid of them.

Eat regularly

When you have a proper food schedule, your body will be able to regulate your blood sugar levels in an efficient fashion. The portions of the meals also matter. Ensure that you do not consume too much during any meal. Here are some pointers to be borne in mind with respect to your meal schedule:

- ➢ Make sure that you start your day with a good breakfast. Not only will this provide you the much needed energy to get on with your schedule but will also help you regulate your blood sugar levels.
- ➢ Another tip to regulate your blood sugar levels is maintaining your calorie intake. Ensure that you consume roughly the same amount of calories every day. Consistency is the key. It is important that your overall calorie intake for each day remains roughly the same as well as the calorie intake for each meal.
- ➢ Keep eating small meals throughout the day. This will again help you regulate your blood sugar levels throughout the day.

Conclusion

I am sure that you would be feeling at ease by now. Diabetes can be quite scaring, especially if you have already seen the effects of it on your friends and family. But do not forget that it can be easily managed, with little efforts and a lot of perseverance from your side. Do not get bogged down by the fact that diabetes runs in the family. We have already seen enough tips in this book to help you avoid diabetes.

Stay focused. Stay grounded. You can definitely manage diabetes just like the zillion things that you are managing on a day to day basis efficiently. I hope you found this book useful and engaging. Thank you again for buying this book. Good luck!

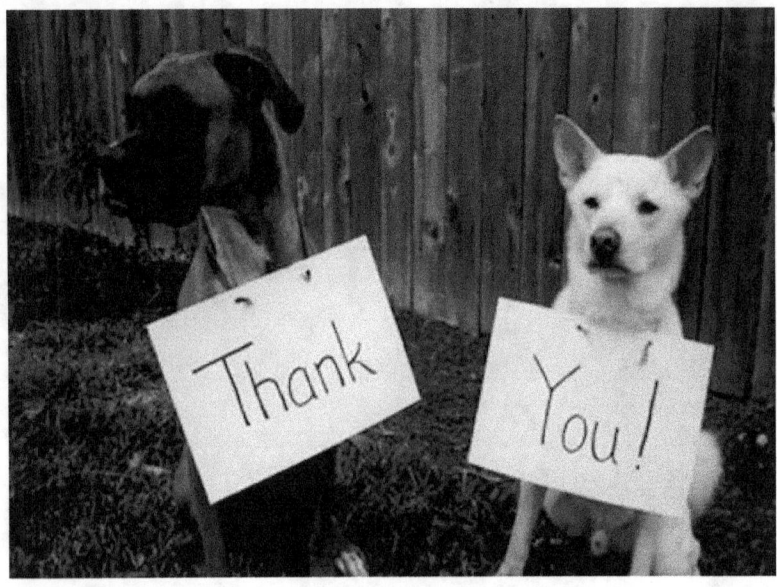

Finally, if you enjoyed this book, then I'd like to ask you for a favour, would you be kind enough to leave a review for this book on Amazon? It'd be greatly appreciated!

!

Chapter 4 – Caring for Organic Vegetables & Fruits

Depending on the plant varieties you choose, your organic vegetable or fruit garden will continue to yield edibles for months at a time. A large variety will also provide a ton of color and beauty.

A lot of the continuing care of your garden will depend on the variety of species you plant. Honestly, your choices are endless, but for brevity's sake, here are care guidelines for some of the more common fruit and veggie choices.

Vegetables

Beans are a popular choice. Green beans are easy to grow and can be harvested throughout the summer and early fall, making them a versatile and long-lasting crop. If space is a concern, grow pole beans. They grow vertically, so will require a stabilizing pole or trellis, but the crop to area ratio is amazing. They also require little in the way of fertilizer since they produce most of the nitrogen they need.

Plant beans in the spring, just after the last frost. The seedlings take well to slightly cooler soil temperatures and they have a growth period of 2-3 months, so start early. They require a moderate amount of sun and water, so special care isn't a necessity with these easy, versatile veggies.

Beets are also quite popular. They come in many varieties, all of which have different tastes and grow periods. Red table beets are by far the most common, as well as the easiest to grow. They do take a while to produce edible roots, so plant these guys a month or so before the last spring frost.

The good news is, they are very hardy. It's actually quite difficult to kill a good crop of beets, so these are a good choice for "black thumbs". They are also very versatile. While the root itself takes several months to reach an edible state, the greens can be harvested as soon as they reach a few inches long. Water them moderately and try to keep them out of harsh sunlight so as not to kill the greens.

For beauty as well as tastiness, why not try cabbage? Whether you choose green or red cabbage, you will be surprised at just how easy they are to grow. Not only are they delicious and nutritious whether cooked or raw, but they are absolutely gorgeous when growing.

One advantage is that you can harvest cabbage twice, once in the spring and again in the fall. These guys love a slight frost toward the end of their growth period, so don't worry about leaving them in the ground too late in the year. They require moderate water, but should be sheltered from too much sun. It is a good idea to do some research on how big each species will grow, and space the seedlings accordingly. Some cabbages can grow to massive proportions, so be careful they don't encroach on each other.

Carrots are always a good choice for a small garden. Chantenay carrots are by far the most popular, as well as one of the easiest to grow. They're the cone-shaped variety you find at the grocery store. Other varieties have different tastes and shapes, but many are a bit picky about where they grow and require a little more dedication.

Plant your carrots early, as they take a few months to get to the edible stage. They're best when planted in the spring, then harvested in summer and fall. The good news is that carrots do well with just about any type of soil, need only a little bit of sun and are fine with moderate watering. Carrots are surprisingly easy to grow and very difficult to kill, making them perfect for a starter garden.

Onions are a staple food around the world, and with so many different varieties, it's easy to find a species that grows perfectly in your climate. There are three types of onions, short-day, intermediate-day and long-day. The types correspond to the length of summer days they grow best in. For example, in the north, summer days last longer sunrise to sunset, so a long-day variety grows quite well.

Once you've chosen your onion variety, it's best to start the seedlings in the winter. Grow them in the house at first, then transfer them to the garden in the spring. These guys absolutely love a lot of sun, so don't be afraid to plant them in the sunniest spot you can find.

Harvest once the tops have fallen, and move them to a dry, shady spot for a few days until they're a little drier and ready to eat.

Peppers are an organic garden's darling. Not only are there a ton of different varieties to choose from, but they are very easy to take care of. You can grow bell peppers, sweet peppers or hot peppers. These will need a stabilizing pole or trellis of some sort, as the plants themselves are long and spindly, while the peppers tend to weigh them down a bit.

Peppers love warm weather, so start the seedlings inside, preferably in the early spring. Grow them until a few weeks after your last frost, then transfer them outside. For a few days before planting them in your garden, let them sit outside for a few hours each day. This way, they will become acclimated to the great outdoors and won't suffer culture shock when transplanted.

Peppers, while easy to care for, do need a lot of sun and water. It's best to keep them separated from root veg, as they require a lot more water and you don't want your carrots getting greedy!

You can harvest peppers as soon as you think they're big enough to eat, though the longer you leave them on the vine the more flavorful and full of vitamins they will be. Dried or pickled peppers will keep a long time, making these an excellent choice for canning.

Tomatoes are one of the most popular choices for home gardening. With so many varieties to choose from (including lovely heirloom types), you're guaranteed to find a species to love. One of the benefits of choosing organically grown tomatoes over the store bought kind is flavor! Store bought tomatoes have typically been genetically modified to look plump and juicy and bright red. Unfortunately, this results in a bland, almost mushy flavor. Your garden-grown tomatoes may not look perfect, but you'll taste the difference with the first bite.

Similar to peppers, you want to start them indoors in the early spring and transplant them around the same time. Acclimatize your tomato plants to the outdoors in the same way.

Because tomatoes need a lot of sun and water, they are great companion plants to peppers. Plant them in the same area and make sure they both get lots of sun and water throughout their growth. Also like peppers, tomatoes can be harvested as soon as you think they're ready, though it's best to leave them on the vine until they are at least a little red!

Fruits

Blueberries are a popular addition to an organic garden. You only need to look at how easily and profusely they grow in the wild to get an idea of how easy it will be to have fresh blueberries in your own garden!

Start blueberries indoors, preferably in the late winter, around January or February. The fruits are small, but the plants themselves need extra time to put down firm roots. Set them out a month or two after initial planting, before the really warm weather hits.

Once your blueberry plant is planted nice and deep and the roots have taken, they really need very little. A sunny patch, a little water and they grow like nobody's business all on their own.

One of the best aspects of growing berries is that they can be left on the bush for quite a while. Pull them off when you want some berries, pop some in your mouth when going about your gardening, and leave the big harvest for late summer. Blueberries are great for preserves and canning, so be sure to save some!

Grapes are a popular choice for trellis coverings, and with a large variety to choose from, it's easy to find one that is perfect for your climate. In general, it's easier to grow grapes in dry climates, but with a little extra care and direct sunlight, grapes can thrive even in humid areas.

For colder climates or those with shorter summers, choose white or green grapes. They ripen more quickly and their thinner skin means they thrive on less heat and sunlight. For longer summers or hotter weather, choose a darker grape. Their thicker skins can handle the intense heat.

Honestly, unless you're going for a prize-winning wine grape, you can grow delicious grapes with little interference. Because they are vine-grown, they do need a fence or trellis to grow along. Natural sunlight and a little water is best, though if you have moderate rain, that's sufficient for their growth. Larger, dark grapes are amazing for jam-making and juicing, while green or white grapes are particularly spectacular when eaten directly off the vine.

Strawberries are one of the most popular home-grown fruits. That's because they bear fruit very easily, are adaptable to different weathers and soil types and taste *so much better* than store bought varieties. Sure, most organically grown fruits and vegetables taste better than the grocery store equivalent, but with strawberries (like tomatoes) the difference is staggering.

For strawberries, it's recommended to start with small plants. You can plant seeds, but keep in mind that it will take one or two years before you start to see any edible fruits. Strawberry plants are not expensive, however, and you can plant seeds every year to have a renewable crop, as one plant will last three or four years by itself.

They love sunny patches, so be sure to keep them out of the shade. Strawberries do well when in the company of other berries, so if you have enough space, think about a mixed berry patch! They have similar growth patterns and needs to blueberries and blackberries, which means you will be up to your elbows in cobblers and jams in no time!

No matter what fruits or vegetables you decide to plant, just be sure that you read directions for planting and pay attention to the individual needs of each species. Once you have a starter garden planted and feel more confident in your gardening abilities, why not try out other, more exotic foods? Heirloom veg are beautiful and often have very unique flavors. Fruit trees, while they are a bit of a time commitment, are a lovely addition to any garden or lawn.

Find out what's best for your climate and soil and plan from there! You can enjoy foods fresh from the garden within a season.

Click HERE To read the full book

Other Books To Read

Below you'll find some other recommended books that are popular on Amazon and Kindle as well. Simply click on the links below to check them out.

Organic Gardening – A beginners step by step guide **by Lisa Shine**

Meditation: Powerful Guide to Meditation in Everyday Life

Cannabis & Cancer: The Medicinal benefits of this miracle herb

If the links do not work, for whatever reason, you can simply search for these titles on the Amazon website to find them.